MY DIRTY LITTLE SECRET

How I Went From Sickness To Health In 120 Days

DR. LEE ANGLE

DEDICATION

This book is written in memory of my mother Karen Angle, who suffered a long and hard battle with cancer which she ultimately lost. She taught me strength in her fight and spurred me to dedicate my life to others, as she had dedicated hers to young minds as a teacher for almost 30 years.

I also want to thank two very special people.

Dr. Perry Rush, the man that gave me my life back through an Upper Cervical correction and taught me how to provide this care to others.

My loving wife Rachel who encouraged me every step of the way.

TABLE OF CONTENTS

INTRODUCTION

I was 31 years old and the picture of health. 245 pounds of muscle, Top 20 in my weight class in the country for powerlifting, I held a state record squat. I ate cleaner than anyone I knew. Underneath it all...I had a dirty little secret. I was physically and mentally broken.

It took me 10 minutes every morning to unfold myself and stand up. Once up, I had to hobble around on crutches for 30-45 minutes until I was able to put weight on my left foot. Otherwise, I would get a pain so severe in my ankle I would at times vomit. This was my daily routine for almost 10 years. I suffered from almost weekly migraines, seemingly endless sinus infections, and more days than not I had burning sciatic pain down my left leg. My digestion was awful. A settled stomach was a rarity. I had incontinence issues that would be sparked by debilitating lower back cramps. That always led to a fun day.

Let's talk about my nighttime routine. I had to put carpal tunnel braces on both hands. You know, the ones with metal in them to keep your hands straight. If I didn't I would wake up sometime during the night feeling like I had dipped my hands in fire. Oh, and that was after I downed some Nyquil just so I could manage to fall asleep. Once all that was squared away about an hour later I would finally doze off.

All of that was just on the physical side. My mental abilities were deteriorating at an even faster pace. I had always been top of my class, a social butterfly, and comfortable in almost any situation. I now found myself on Zoloft for my depression and anxiety, with OCD which wouldn't allow me to use a toothbrush more than once or step on a crack on a sidewalk. I felt like I was losing my mind and my body was almost gone.

At this point, I had nearly given up on the idea of a happy successful life. It was just a race to see which fully collapsed first, my brain or my body. I had tried medications, I tried therapy, I even went to chiropractors for years. I ate like an Olympic athlete and exercised like a madman yet there I was, feeling close to hopeless.

Around that time a man named Dr. Perry Rush entered my life. He told me about a bone in my neck that could be the source of all of my issues. Naturally, I thought he was crazy, but as I was out of options I kept listening. He went through the philosophy, history, and practice of what he referred to as Upper Cervical Chiropractic. I had tried chiropractic for many years but what he described seemed very different. I finally decided I might as well give it a shot. I was in a "what do I have to lose" position.

I began the Upper Cervical process (a process I will explain throughout this book) hopeful but with reservations. Everything else I had tried failed me and I suspected this might work out the same.

My x-rays revealed a significant amount of damage in my neck. A surprising amount for my age, but I also welcomed some actual visual evidence which might explain some of my issues. I received my first adjustment. The top bone in my neck was misaligned and Dr. Rush returned it to its normal position. I didn't realize it but my life would never be the same following that adjustment. It seemed like a small maneuver but it really changed the course of my life.

Over the following weeks, I noticed I could actually sleep. My hands still had some tingling but the terrible burning at night was gone. I could eat without my stomach feeling terrible for hours afterward. My anxiety level was down considerably and my ability to think and make quick decisions was starting to return. My hip and back pain was still present but, that began when I was 14 years old and ended up being the last thing to leave. A few months in I almost felt like a new person. The mental issues which had been growing over the last few years had pretty much disappeared and my body felt like it was finally working again. Within 120 days I felt like a new person. I had endless energy, I enjoyed being around friends and family again, and I felt like I could take on the world.

That first adjustment was in 2006. I still have an occasional ache or pain, but my overall well-being has dramatically improved. I quickly decided I wanted to provide this same care so others could experience what I had and live a better life as I now do.

I have practiced Upper Cervical Chiropractic since 2009 and have been privileged to see patient after patient experience life-changing results just like mine. With each passing year, I still can't believe how great I feel after suffering for so long. I had deteriorated to a recluse with chronic pain and now have a successful practice, a wonderful family and the honor of caring for others. I owe it all to that first adjustment.

The purpose and motivation for this book is to share my "dirty little secret" with as many people as possible. That is the reason why I feel significantly years younger than I did at 31. The reason my health, and in turn my life, has been restored and improved upon daily. The power of a proper adjustment at the proper time can have further reaching implications than you have likely ever experienced. That is the power of life being restored!

In the words of the late Dr. B.J. Palmer, the developer of Chiropractic and the founder of Upper Cervical, "Have you more faith in a spoonful of medicine than in the power that animates the living world?". In other words...

I want to show you how this power can be unlocked in you and allow your health and life to be restored.

CHAPTER 1

WHAT IS UPPER CERVICAL CHIROPRACTIC?

Before we begin let's come to a couple of agreements First, I will use as little doctor speak as possible if you agree to stick with me where technical points can't be avoided. Second, I promise to not give you anything I can't back up, if you promise to keep an open mind, no matter what you previously thought about chiropractic. Now that we have that out of the way, let's answer the big question. What is Upper Cervical Chiropractic?

Upper cervical refers to the top two bones in your spine, right where your head meets your body. These two bones are special for several reasons. They are the only vertebrae with names, indicating they're in fact quite different than any of the other bones in your spine...

The top bone is the atlas.

The second, the axis.

Remember Atlas from Greek mythology, Carrying the weight of the world atop his shoulders? Well, your atlas supports your whole world: Your brain. This single bone weighs about 2 ounces, meanwhile, the average head weighs 10-12 pounds.

And the second bone, the axis? Well,here's the definition of any old axis:

noun, plural ax·es [ak-seez] /'æk siz/.

the line about which a rotating body, such as the earth, turns

So as you might guess, your world rotates on this axis, a single, tiny bone at the top of your neck.

These are also the smallest bones in the spine along with being the most freely moveable. This allows us to move our head in ways the rest of the spine cannot but also sets us up for injury. With more mobility comes more instability.

Now that we have the names and stats out of the way, forget about the bones. Wait.....what? Ok, don't forget about them, but what they surround and protect is the real star of our story. The brainstem. Our brain is in our skull and the lower portion of the brain is the brainstem. It starts in the skull and extends down into the atlas and axis, (also known as C1 and C2) the top two bones in the neck. The brainstem is the first bundle of tissues that develops after conception and everything else that makes us, grows out of it. With this development, our entire body is connected by nerves which allow our brain and body to communicate. The brainstem is the central hub of this system and the key component which enables our bodies to function.

A healthy brainstem gives us a high potential for a healthy body. A compromised brainstem can lead to big problems with our health. The health of the brainstem is partly determined by the proper positioning and movement of those top 2 bones. Proper diet, proper exercise and stress all play a role in health, but without a properly functioning nervous system, you won't reap the full benefits. Your body won't be able to digest and absorb food properly or manage stress nearly as easily.

Most people see chiropractic as all about the bones. That is the large disconnect between the public and the profession. As you learn what I know, you will see the power of a proper adjustment at the proper place and time is crucial in finding whole body wellness. In the coming chapters, I will share this knowledge with you so you can unlock the healthiest version of yourself like I did. I want to connect you to the real "why" of chiropractic and specifically the brand of Upper Cervical chiropractic. By the time you finish reading this book, I am pretty certain we will be on the same page if not, at least I dressed up for the cover photo and the book will look good on your shelf.

If you are like I was, you may think Chiropractic is a pretty reasonable way to take care of some back and neck pain, maybe a headache. If that is you, I would like to apologize to you for my profession. I want to apologize because you were misled. This profession promotes help for neck and back pain, for musculoskeletal conditions. Chiropractic isn't always taught as a means to a healthy nervous system which allows your body to function properly, to heal, to be all that It can be. We were told, if you play a game of pick up basketball and get knocked around or had a fall you should come in and get adjusted.

It wasn't the medical doctors that misled you, it wasn't "big pharma" or anyone else. I am sad to say it was the profession of Chiropractic. That isn't a blanket statement as there are chiropractors who teach the truth. The profession as a whole, however, has somewhat lost its way. The unified message of chiropractic has been false, powerless, and to me downright infuriating. The reasons are various from trying to satisfy insurance companies, attempting to gain acceptance from the medical community and looking to fill some void that did not need to be filled. Is it any surprise the average person is missing out on the big picture of chiropractic when so much of the profession is missing out?

It's certainly not your fault. We all believe what we're told or believe what we're shown if we are told and shown enough. If my entire life I had been told that toothpaste was to wash my hair then I guess I would be washing my hair with toothpaste. It would be a terrible way to do it, but if that's how the product was marketed, that is likely how I would use it. I would be missing the bigger purpose of cleaning my teeth so they wouldn't rot and decay. It might even harm your hair, things done improperly can cause damage.

Chiropractic did not begin as a treatment for back pain, in fact, the first patient was a man who had a neck injury and lost his hearing. Seventeen years later he was adjusted and his hearing returned. From that time forward chiropractic was practiced, researched, and marketed as a method to restore the proper brain to body communication, allowing the body to heal from about anything. Then chiropractic entered the dark ages. The eighties came along with insurance reimbursements. It was much easier to tell the insurance company we were correcting back and neck pain than correcting nervous system interference. Suddenly chiropractic became the back crack shack (that was the actual name of a clinic near one of my practices…..). the message of musculoskeletal conditions started to be sold because, quite frankly, that's what the insurance would pay for.

Thankfully the profession is coming back out of the Dark Ages. Insurance reimbursements aren't what they used to be and with the greater sharing of knowledge from the internet, the real message is starting to get out again. The philosophy is being put back in and as a result, we see more and more chiropractors graduating every day who are practicing real Chiropractic with real power. Teaching their patients and communities what it can truly be. Just to be clear, I'm not saying it's not great for back pain, neck pain and headaches. In my testimonial at the beginning of this book, I discussed how Chiropractic rid me of those things. BUT remember all the other things? It isn't voodoo or black magic, it is physiology. It will all make sense once I lay a little groundwork.

I grew up watching westerns. Saturday mornings were for cowboys and the open prairie. Hondo, Gunsmoke, Wagon Train, and Branded were my cartoons. If you watch westerns long enough you inevitably see the wagon rolling into town selling potions and lotions. The "snake oil" salesmen of the west. A guy would jump out of his sign covered wagon, hold up his bottle of ointment, and promise to heal anyone in earshot of anything that ailed them. Most sales presentations ended the same for the snake oil salesman. Either the sheriff would come by and tell him to move on or some ruffian in the crowd would threaten to shoot him on the spot.

A quick glance at most chiropractic marketing, especially Upper Cervical, and you may feel like the snake oil wagon has driven into town. You will see a variety of conditions that have responded positively to UC adjustments. From pain to diabetes, and even things like multiple sclerosis. The first thought for some is how is that possible and for others, it seems like a scam. I get it, but once we piece it together it will start to make a lot of sense. Once you have a base understanding of how our incredible bodies work it all becomes very clear and makes perfect sense how one thing can contribute to so many problems.

CHAPER 2

DON'T RIDE THE BRAKES

A sk a group of people what's the first thing that develops after con-ception, the majority answer the heart. We think of our heart as the most important, the master of the body. We check blood pressure and pulse rate. We worry about heart attacks, cholesterol numbers and all sorts of gauges to make sure our heart is healthy throughout our life-time. While our heart is certainly important and necessary, it is neither the first thing that develops nor the most important.

The first thing that develops after conception is the brainstem. After it develops to some degree, the brain grows out of the top, the spinal cord out of the bottom and then spinal nerves. Our organs, tissues, and mus-cles grow from the spinal nerves. This allows our entire body to be con-nected. Our wiring system, which we call the nervous system, can now transfer information and direct the development process to form a func-tioning body.

Once the nervous system is fully developed and we have a formed per-son, the function and health of that person is largely determined by the function and health of the nervous system. When we break that system into two parts, the picture starts to become clearer. Technically speaking you have the sympathetic and parasympathetic nervous system.

Think about a time you were in danger or really stressed, or about to take a game-winning shot. What happens? Your pulse goes up, your blood pressure goes up, your awareness goes up, all of your senses are on edge. This gas pedal on our body is the work of the sympathetic nerv-ous system. This is known as our fight or flight response.

Now, think about a time when you were incredibly relaxed. You just had a great meal, the lights are down and you start getting a little sleepy. Everything feels like it's moving slower. Your pulse is slower, blood pressure drops, muscles feel looser and your whole body feels a little like Jell-O. It feels like the brakes have been applied. This is the work of the parasympathetic nervous system also known as the Rest and Digest response.

These two systems are both working 100% of the time. There is always some gas pedal and always some brake. One system will always be dominant depending on the situation. Please don't go drive your car this way. If I see you going down the road 50 miles an hour with your brake lights continuously on I'm going to be a little worried. In our body the gas/brake combo is necessary, it creates balance. This balance is what we need to have situation appropriate blood pressure, proper hormone levels, just the right amount of enzymes, neurotransmitters and literally a billion other things. These billions of functions also have to occur at the exact moment in an exact sequence. The best part is, all of this is done without conscious thought. You can certainly alter this momentarily by getting yourself worked up or sitting quietly taking deep breaths or meditating but in general, this is going on all the time without us really thinking about it.

Here is the problem. If we get in a situation where the gas pedal is pushed down and dominates for too long we get in trouble. The same goes for the brake.

Let me give you two extreme examples of patients I've helped and then we will discuss the more average cases.

I'll start with a patient whose brake pedal was shoved through the bottom of the car.

When I first sit down with a patient I review their paperwork but I like to discuss their history. I generally lead with "tell me the story". Most everyone has a story about how they end up in the office and I want to get as much information as I can. Remember, my job goes beyond the pain they are feeling. The more information I have the more I can help. The story Susan told was unlike anything I had heard or have heard since. For almost 10 years she had been nearly bedridden. If she drank more than a bottle cap of liquid at a time she would "pass out" for four hours. I used quotation marks because pass out isn't exactly what would happen. She would be motionless and couldn't move but could still hear and was aware.....but unable to move at all. Can you imagine? She had barely left her house during this time and life had passed her by.

When she would eat more than something the equivalent size of a cracker the same thing would happen. Her rest or digest side would attack so hard she had what is known as a freeze response. Her body would just cease to move. Countless doctor visits and medications had made no improvements.

She came to my office as a last resort knowing an accident that injured her neck had occurred before all of this started. Hoping that her neck was the key to her struggle.

After she told me this incredible story we did an Upper Cervical exam and took x rays. I found a very large misalignment of the top bone in her neck (C1). I corrected it that day and over the next several month's something amazing happened. The body that had become her prison was finally set free. She was able to eat almost normally, she could leave the house and go out in the world. That December she attended Christmas with her family for the first time in 10 years! Correcting the misalignment of that top bone took the pressure off her brainstem and allowed the brake/gas balance to be restored.

Now, let's look at someone with the gas pedal mashed down.

Have you ever met someone who looks like they haven't slept in a week yet they are running around a thousand miles an hour? That is how

Donna looked and felt when she came in on day one. She told me that she usually slept a total of 3 hours a night in 15-minute bouts. The rest of the night was tossing and turning, staring at the ceiling. She had high blood pressure, severe anxiety, and endless fatigue. Her digestion was terrible, flipping back and forth from diarrhea to constipation. When I asked when was the last time she didn't have a headache she couldn't remember. "Maybe when I was 5 or 6".

Her immune system was terrible and she was sick more often than not. Again, we did an exam and took x rays. I found a misalignment of both the top (c1) and the second bone (c2) in her neck. Once corrected the gas pedal let up and she began to improve almost immediately. Her digestive issues disappeared almost instantly, her immune system began to fight again, and her overall anxiety level decreased dramatically. She was able to sleep through the night and get off her blood pressure medication. Again, life was restored.

Both of these are more extreme examples but they give you an idea of what can happen when a body gets out of balance.

Autonomic nervous system (ANS) imbalance, like Susan and Donna, is just one of the possible outcomes of an upper cervical misalignment. Complications can be separated into 4 categories ANS dysfunction, Cerebrospinal fluid flow, direct nerve pressure and decreased blood flow to the brain.

These overlap in most cases but we will look at the possible result of each.

CHAPTER 3

ANS DYSFUNCTION

We looked at two extreme cases in Susan and Donna. Most fall somewhere in the middle of those two. The biggest reason for all of this is something called the Vagus nerve. For many years Upper Cervical doctors delivered incredible results but couldn't always explain why.

When I was first in practice, I had a patient who was dealing with extreme constipation. I asked Melissa how often she went to the bathroom. Her answer shocked me. She said an average of once per week. Can you imagine? If that wasn't bad enough, the answer to my next question blew my mind. How long has it been since you went currently? 28 DAYS...that's right 28 days! As you would imagine she was in pain, her body was toxic, and as a result, she was on a number of medications to combat both the constipation and the symptoms stemming from it.

I examined her upper neck and found evidence of a misalignment. X-rays were taken and I found the top bone in her neck (C1) shoved backward and rotated to the left. I asked her about traumas over the years and it turns out (as it so often does) she had a trauma. She had been in an auto accident a few months before the constipation began. I adjusted her and within 10 minutes she ran to the bathroom. That was the end of her constipation issues. Not just for the day but for good.

I knew it happened. I had witnessed all sorts of digestive issues clear up in patients over and over. I just didn't, at the time, fully understand the answer was specifically the vagus nerve. It is known as the tenth cranial nerve (we will discuss some of the other cranial nerves later) This incredibly important nerve starts in our brainstem and travels down the length of most of our upper body. It can be argued that it is the most important nerve in our body as it branches off to our esophagus, heart, lungs, and digestive tract. The vagus nerve is the key to our braking system. It delivers slow down messages to all of these organs.

We discussed that the body has to have balance between the gas (sympathetic) and brake (parasympathetic). The way our bodies find balance is the gas is always pushed and it is the job of the vagus nerve to apply just enough slow down impulses and keep everything in check. If the vagus isn't sending enough impulses, our body speeds up, without any regulation to maintain a healthy balance. This is when our bodies malfunction.

If the vagus is underactive it can lead to:

- high blood pressure
- Fibrillations
- throat spasms
- the lung constriction in asthma
- Diarrhea

If the vagus is overactive the body goes the other direction.

- Low blood pressure
- Fainting
- constipation
- difficulty swallowing
- depression
- Bloating

These are both small lists of the possible outcomes but you get the idea. These outcomes make a lot of sense now that we know the vagus nerve controls organs that are associated with these disorders. Now, here is the even bigger picture. The nervous system, the immune system, and the endocrine system (hormones) are all tightly linked together. I won't go down the rabbit hole of how they are all intertwined but it is safe to say if the vagus nerve is malfunctioning so will the immune and endocrine systems. In other words, we won't be able to fight off infection, viruses, or self heal nearly as efficiently if at all in extreme cases. Hormone imbalance is a book in itself but I will touch on it in another chapter as so many people deal with it on a daily basis.

So the question remains, how do those first two bones affect this important nerve.

The vagus nerve passes through the upper neck before it travels down the spine and exits at different levels. In the case of most, trauma has occurred to misalign the bone(s) and put pressure on the vagus as it travels through. This pressure causes the nerve to malfunction. As with anything in our bodies, it is a bit more complex but I promised to keep the doctor talk to a minimum and you are likely growing tired of me saying vagus.....so grab a cup of coffee (unless you already have too much gas pedal) and take a quick break.

CHAPTER 4

BRAIN HEALTH

The second possible malfunction coming from a UC misalignment is the flow of cerebrospinal fluid. Our brains need a few things to be healthy. Water, glucose (a form of sugar), blood flow, cerebrospinal fluid (the brains padding and nutrient transport fluid), and input from the rest of the body. If it is lacking in any of these, "Houston we have a problem". Those of you old enough will understand that reference, those of you that are younger watch Apollo 13. Tom Hanks is, as always, fantastic. In any case, the brain isn't going to function up to par.

Have you ever been dehydrated? You have a headache, it is hard to think clearly and it feels like you are just off. What about an extreme diet or fast? Your blood sugar drops and you just want to go to bed or bite someone's head off. The brain is low on glucose and goes into survival mode to some extent.

Maintaining water and glucose intake are really your job. Like most jobs the better you do it the better the result will be. My job comes in when we talk about blood flow, cerebrospinal fluid (CSF), and input from the body. All of those can be deeply impacted by the positioning of the upper neck bones.

The vertebral arteries which deliver about 25% of the brain's blood supply, run through the top 4 bones in the neck. There are two vertebral arteries, one on the left one on the right. Once they exit the top bone (C1 or Atlas) they weave around and enter the skull. Mechanical pressure from a rotation of the top bone can close off one of these arteries. Suddenly the brain isn't getting sufficient blood flow. That is never good in any situation, right? The same is true here.

Vertebral artery compression can lead to:

- visual disturbances (double vision, loss of vision)
- weakness or tingling
- loss of balance
- dizziness or vertigo
- brain fog
- difficulty swallowing
- weakness in any part of the body

As you can see compression to these arteries can have a major impact on your quality of life. Luckily it doesn't require surgery or invasive procedures. It just requires restoring the vertebrae in the neck to their proper position and relieving the pressure on the artery which restores the proper blood flow.

Now, let's compound the issue with CSF. CSF is made in the brain then travels out of the skull into the spinal column. It is vital for brain and spinal health. It serves several purposes. It pads and protects the brain and spinal cord, it provides nutrients and takes away waste. Proper flow rate and pressure are key.

Have you heard of hydrocephalus? It is a condition where a baby will have "water on the brain" and swelling coming out of their head. This "water" and swelling is CSF. The reason the head is able to swell is the bones in a newborn's head aren't fused together yet. In healthy children, this enables them to exit the birth canal and look a bit like a cone head when they first come out. As we grow and develop these bones fuse into the hard case of bone we think of as our skull.

Remember CSF is constantly made in your brain. A certain pressure is kept in the skull the rest drains out of the head and down the spinal column. It drains kind of like a sink with one main drain that also has a number of small drains in it. If the small drains get clogged the main drain struggles to keep up and we get water pooling. The same thing can happen in the skull. The small drains get blocked and CSF begins to pool. The skull is hard bone, the only other option is for the fluid to start squeezing the brain. This squeeze makes it more difficult for nerves to carry messages and blood to flow.

This can lead to:

- Headaches
- Blurred vision
- Nausea
- Seizures
- Difficulty walking
- Fatigue
- Issues with memory/brain fog

This list could keep going but the consequences should be clear. Multiple Sclerosis has also been linked to the pooling of CSF. It leeches off elements that can damage the brain and produce the trademark plaquing seen in MS.

Once again, just like with the vertebral arteries, we are dealing with a mechanical pressure issue. One of the upper neck bones (primarily C1) gets misaligned due to a trauma and compresses one or more of the accessory drainage pathways and the fluid begins to pool in the head. When we correct the misalignment the fluid flow is restored and the issues typically disappear.

That leaves us with the last component the brain needs to function properly. This is a big one. Input from the rest of the body. Did you know it has been estimated that 90% of brain development in an infant/toddler is from body movement. It is the fuel that allows the brain to grow. It isn't a coincidence that babies start walking before they start really talking. As we grow we begin to get brain stimulation from language, visual input, and other stimulus, but proper development is largely based on movement. Babies are constantly wiggling around and moving their arms and legs. This movement drives the brain and gives it vital input.

All of this input enters the brainstem and is then transferred to the brain. As I said earlier the brainstem is our main communication hub. If the brainstem is compromised, so too will the input to the brain be compromised. If the brain lacks proper input the development will inevitably suffer. An upper cervical misalignment can distort this input.

I will tell you my favorite story to date after seeing thousands of patients. I often tell this story when I give talks. I have yet to get through it without a few tears.

A 4-year-old young man named Riley was brought to me by his very loving and very concerned parents. Riley had been diagnosed with autism. He had all of the classic signs. No eye contact, he did not like to be touched and he was very limited verbally. He was still eating baby food (he gagged on anything else) and in a diaper. During the consult, he ran in circles yelling for 20 minutes and crashing into my window blinds. This first visit was purely fact-finding. I had them bring him by a few more times until he was comfortable enough with me to do an exam.

The exam revealed he had a reverse curvature in his neck (more on spinal curves later) and the top bone (C1) in his neck was very far forward. Thermography showed a lot of pressure at the top of his neck. I explained my findings to his parents and we set out to correct his neck and see what happened.

The next few months shocked me (I had only been in practice a few months at this point). I expected improvements, I understood the mechanisms that were in play and I still sat back in awe of what happened. Within 2 months Riley was potty trained, he could eat anything, he would walk into the office, look me right in the eye and tell me what he had done that day. Now let's play "I'm not crying you're crying". His mom walked in one day and gave me a giant hug. Riley had hugged her and told her he loved her for the first time ever. He had always shown it in other ways but for him to be able to express it in words was very special for all of us.

I have to tell you that experience changed me. My personal experience had affirmed my faith in the procedure and driven my desire to provide this service to others. Riley's transformation turbocharged it and solidified the power of proper Upper Cervical chiropractic care.

Not every single case is this miraculous but I have seen such incredible results in so many kids, I believe it should be standard procedure for all children to be checked, just to be certain their necks are in good alignment and nerve system is working at 100%

Think about it, it isn't always easy to get into the world. Forceps, suction, C-sections, long deliveries where the doctor has to really pull to get the baby out. All of these are hard on a tiny neck with no muscle strength to protect the structures.

Then as a child begins to walk they fall all over the place and once they learn to walk all bets are off. Head into tables, doors, falling backwards and banging their heads. It is endless.

I have seen several studies touting how common this issue is in newborns and children. Like all studies, if you look hard enough you can likely poke a few holes in them. So, I don't like to throw out percentages. What I will say is that it happens, I see it happen daily.

I have children come in with colic, digestive issues, skin conditions, autism, fevers, poor immune function and so much more. I adjust them and they get better. Restoration to normal function happens consistently. Because for a child who can't properly explain or voice what is wrong all we see is their reactions. Chiropractic exams can reveal the unseen issues.

It is worth the short time investment to have them checked. If they are aligned, no one will be happier than the Upper Cervical doctor, if they are not, it is much easier to fix a problem at the beginning than later down the road. When you restore function you are allowing normal development to be restored as well. Children are constantly developing and their un-coordinated, wiggy bodies can do damage that goes unnoticed if not properly monitored. This isn't just for kids with signs of autism, this is for the proper function and development of everything and everyone with a spine.

CHAPTER 5

DIRECT NERVE PRESSURE

S ome conditions aren't all that complicated. They don't involve a precise sync of multiple parts of the brain, they don't rely on a perfectly timed cascade of hormones. There is simply a nerve that is being compressed and causing terrible pain. If pain isn't the result it is either significant weakness, numbness/tingling or itching. Some of these cases have a named diagnosis. Trigeminal neuralgia and Occipital Neuralgia are things we see in an upper cervical office frequently and have great results.

The spine is a complex system of parts but is fairly simple in its design. 24 individual bones stacked on top of each other with a joint in between. At each level a nerve exits on the left and a nerve exits on the right. Each nerve has a destination. Some go to muscles, others to organs, etc. All of these nerves branch off the spinal cord. The spinal cord (and as a result all nerves) begins at the brain/brainstem. A nerve can be compressed at any point between the brain and its destination.

Think about a phone line (remember those…). If I cut it as it enters the phone or as it leaves the pole the result is the same right? Communication is interrupted regardless of where the interference occurs.

The main causes of nerve compression are a spinal disc bulge, arthritis, disc degeneration, and spinal misalignment. Have you heard the term stenosis? If you have ever had a spinal MRI you may have seen the words "spinal canal stenosis" or "foraminal stenosis". Stenosis simply means a space has gotten smaller. Take your hand and touch your thumb with your index and middle finger. There is a round space created. Now pinch your fingers together a bit. See how it closes the space down? That is stenosis. If the space where a nerve travels closes down it can cause mechanical pressure. If the pressure is severe enough this is what you think of as a pinched nerve. Motor nerves compressed will lead to weakness, pain nerves will deliver pain and sensory nerves will give you numbness/tingling.

The longer there is pressure the more damage there will be to the nerve. In these cases, symptoms generally get worse with time. The traditional treatment route is a referral to physical therapy. In some cases this works but in others, there is either no benefit or it makes things worse. If you are trying to move, stretch, and exercise a set of bones that aren't moving properly it often aggravates the system.

If PT fails the next move is usually pain management. Injections are given to try to eliminate or at least diminish the pain. Again, sometimes it works, sometimes it doesn't. Either way, the original issue wasn't corrected, you just don't feel it anymore. What do you do now? Often overdue or stress the area and do more damage. Once the injection wears off it is worse than ever.

Now we are in a position where surgery is being discussed. Sometimes the damage is so severe, surgery is the only option. In those cases, I am glad there are dedicated, skilled surgeons that can stabilize the area and remove the pressure.

In most cases, the real issue is a loss of biomechanics. The spine gets misaligned and as a result it loses the proper movement and gets stiff. This eventually leads to a loss of the proper curve and now the pressure on the discs and bones is much greater. Eventually, the soft tissue of a disc begins to degenerate or it bulges out. Either of these can lead to nerve pressure. If the bones have extra pressure on them long enough they get inflamed. The body responds by building extra bone. This results in bone spurs. As that bone grows the space for the nerves decreases.

In these cases, restoring the proper alignment and movement to the spine can begin to undo the damage. This takes the pressure off the nerves. As they begin to heal the symptoms will begin to decrease. Remember I had to wear braces on my wrists every night for years? The nerves in my neck were getting crushed from disc degeneration and some pretty nasty bone spurs. My neck was stiff and locked into a bad position. Once the top bone in my neck was corrected and my head was on straight, my neck began to loosen up and the pressure was taken off of the nerves. I was able to throw the braces away and haven't had any burning in my hands for a very long time.

Degeneration and bone spurs aren't always a life sentence. Mine were rough in my early 30s but are much smaller and I do not have any issues with them now. It just takes time and proper care to allow the body to correct and heal itself.

CHAPTER 6

CAN THIS AFFECT MY HORMONES?

Believe it or not, people are not always happy with positive results. I walked into my front desk area one day and heard a young lady say that she would not be back. She seemed a bit upset. I asked her if she would step into my office and explain the issue. Naturally, I thought she might be unhappy with her care, billing, or some sort of misunderstanding. Her answer to why she was upset and would not be returning left me almost speechless. She told me that prior to seeing me she only had a period once or twice a year. Now that the pressure was off her brainstem and her body was working correctly, she had a period every month and "that is just too much aggravation and work". We discussed that was the natural order of things but she knowingly chose for her body to malfunction. I shook my head and wished her well. I was happy that her body was healthy, but her choices were her own.

The natural question here is how does adjusting the neck affect menstrual cycles?

The nervous system, the endocrine system, and the immune system are all tightly linked and the function of one will influence another. The endocrine system is responsible for all of our hormones. Whether those are for reproduction, emotion, or the massive list of other functions of hormones provide.

Let's start with the menstrual cycle. There are hormones to start it, continue it, and stop it. The timing and amounts are vital. Too much of one hormone and not enough of another and the whole thing starts to fall apart.

I have a small section on my intake form that asks about menstruation. Is it regular, painful (abnormally), and have they had miscarriages. More often than not something is not "normal". So many women spend half the month miserable. Jokes are made about PMS but it can genuinely be a real problem for some. Depression, difficulty functioning, and even suicidal thoughts in extreme cases. Once it begins severe cramps, clotting, and endometriosis can make it difficult to get through the day. Imagine dealing with that month in and month out.

Most turn to birth control pills to try to better regulate. Like all medications, these have side effects and for those that would like to, conception is not a possibility. On that topic, if this cycle isn't properly balanced hormonally, the chances of conception are very low. I have had a number of patients who failed to conceive and once we restored function and their cycle normalized they were able to get pregnant. I am not saying that Upper Cervical Chiropractic is the only answer for infertility but I will say ask any UC doc and they will have more than a handful of stories with the same result. This makes sense as we begin to see how the body fits together. When we open the pathway to proper communication we are allowing the body a chance to self regulate. Balanced hormones is something we can all see the value in.

The menstrual cycle starts with a signal from the hypothalamus (a vital section of our brain) to the pituitary gland to secrete follicle-stimulating hormone which then travels to the ovaries to start the process. If the hypothalamus fails to send this signal or it just isn't right the hormone level begins to be altered. The end result is no cycle at all or an abnormal cycle.

The hypothalamus gets most of its input from...you guessed it the brainstem. The upper cervical spine protects the lower portion of the brainstem. A misalignment puts pressure on the brainstem and causes the input to the hypothalamus to be incorrect. Garbage in, garbage out applies here. Bad input equals bad output and the body malfunctions. If the hypothalamus over or under stimulates the pituitary we fall into a hormone imbalance.

The link between the hypothalamus and the pituitary gland is incredibly important when discussing hormone imbalances and issues. The pituitary gland is responsible for most hormone functions and is often called the master gland.

The pituitary gland is responsible for:

- Thyroid hormones
- Reproductive hormones
- Stress hormones
- Growth hormone
- Hormones responsible for blood pressure
- Hormones responsible for metabolism

This list is just direct pituitary function not even counting the influence on other glands. If it is stimulated to secrete too much or too little you can see how a great number of things can go wrong.

I know I promised at the beginning to keep the technical talk to a minimum but if you get an idea of how it all works, you begin to see the real influence.

Thyroid issues are incredibly common. A few years ago it was a trend to chop them out either fully or partially. Thankfully that has decreased significantly. Sometimes surgery is the only answer but it should be a last resort after dietary changes are made and structural neurological integrity is evaluated and restored. I won't go through the pathway again (you are welcome) but the pituitary directly influences the thyroid. Bad pituitary function = bad thyroid function.

Before you elect for surgery or medication make sure your diet is on point and your head is on straight.

Hormones aren't just for women. When a man has a hormonal imbalance it can lead to all sorts of issues. Low energy, low libido, some types of cancer, mood issues and an increased cardiovascular risk. These are just a few of the many possible outcomes for men. Women's hormones get most of the attention and press, but many men struggle daily with hormone issues that have never been addressed and are often avoidable. The effects can be devastating. Failed marriages, low productivity, and a lack of enjoyment of life. I have so many men come in as patients and tell me they have little energy, no motivation, and a lack of interest in sex. These issues are often chalked up to aging, but once they have their upper neck corrected and life begins to flow, they begin to wake up with energy and a desire to live fully again.

CHAPTER 7

WHAT ABOUT MENTAL HEALTH?

The teen depression rate is alarming and their suicide rate is terrifying. In fact, according to suicide.org, a teen takes his or her own life every 100 minutes. Suicide is the third-leading cause of death for young people ages 15 to 24. Approximately 20% of teens experience depression before they reach adulthood, and between 10% to 15% suffer from depression symptoms at any one time.

The latest statistics from 2017 report:

- 300 million people around the world have depression, according to the World Health Organization
- 17.3 million adults in the United States—equaling 7.1 percent of all adults in the country—have experienced a major depressive episode in the past year
- 11 million U.S. adults experienced an episode that resulted in severe mental impairment in the past year
- Nearly 50 percent of all people diagnosed with depression are also diagnosed with an anxiety disorder
- It's estimated that 15 percent of the adult population will experience depression at some point in their lifetime.

Depression is a complex topic. The potential causes vary widely and include abuse, genetics, social pressures, and more. External factors can certainly play a big role but many who suffer from depression or anxiety will tell you they "don't really have anything to be upset about" but cannot seem to get on the other side of feeling depressed. On the other hand, things may not be great but the feelings still do not match the situation. If circumstances do not match up with emotion then we have to look internally. Proper brain communication and hormone balance becomes the focus. Let's look at the brain first.

Multiple areas of the brain have been shown to decrease in size and/or activity in depressed individuals and other areas are more active. If areas that spark negative emotions are overstimulated and areas that bring joy are understimulated consistently we have a big problem. When something bad occurs it is natural for the negative emotions to be generated. If they are being generated all the time due to a physiological problem then life will begin to feel terrible all the time. The lack of joy from a reward or from things going well just compounds the feeling that everything is awful and there is no hope in sight.

First, let's look at the difference in a teen brain compared to an adult. One of the biggest differences is the development of the prefrontal cortex. The prefrontal cortex is responsible for rational thought. This area isn't fully developed until around age 25. This area of the brain allows us to consider consequences, think before we act, and better control inappropriate behaviors. Studies suggest that teens make decisions that are more driven by the amygdala. This is important because the amygdala is the heart of our emotional system. So when a teen over-reacts or gets highly emotional at situations in a way that seems irrational, this difference is what is at play.

The amygdala (I know this is getting sciency but stick with me, and it will soon make sense) is important for the processing of emotions, especially negative emotions. This includes fear, anger, panic, and anxiety. The more the amygdala is stimulated, the greater these emotions will be felt. Much of the stimulus of the amygdala comes from our senses, all the information the body collects from our eyes, ears, and skin. This is part of our fight or flight response. If we are in a calm and safe environment, the amygdala and these emotions should, in theory, be calm and relaxed.

All of this sensory information is gathered, then sent to the brainstem. The brainstem is at the base of our brain and extends into the upper cervical part of our neck between the top two vertebrae. The brainstem takes this information and sends it to the Thalamus, (which is basically a relay center which sends information to multiple parts of the brain) which then sends the sensory information to the amygdala.

Now, let's tie this all together. If the sensory information from the body reaches the amygdala properly, then we will have the appropriate emotions and feelings for the environment and situation we are currently experiencing. If, however, this information is distorted, it can overstimulate the amygdala, and now we have negative emotions that do not fit with our situation. If one of the top two bones in the neck is misaligned, it can place mechanical pressure on the brainstem. This pressure irritates the nerves and has the ability to distort the information they carry. Our brain is then getting inaccurate information, and problems begin.

Not every case of teen depression or suicide can be explained by this being the problem, and as I said at the beginning, it is a multi-factor issue. Correcting the upper neck is not always the answer, but it certainly could be. Having this area evaluated is an important piece of the puzzle for teens who are struggling.

I had a concerned mom bring her 14-year-old daughter to see me. Let's call her Anne. Anne had struggled from depression since she was 11. She was once a happy and socially-engaging girl who became a reclusive and angry young teen. She was on multiple medications and had begun to cut herself on her worst days. She was no longer in school because she had such severe anxiety she could barely leave the house. Anne was angry at the world and had attempted to kill herself twice over the last six months. Many hours of therapy, and attempt after attempt with different medications had made almost no difference at all.

I found a rather large misalignment of the top bone in her neck (C1 or Atlas). Over the next two months, we monitored her neck and adjusted it when necessary. The transformation was readily apparent. She stopped cutting almost immediately. Anne started helping out around the house more and began having fun with her family again. She told me she no longer felt like she didn't want to live, and she began to think about her future in a positive light.

This was back in 2012, and I am happy to say she returned to school, graduated, attended college, and is now in a career and doing great. Her depression and anxiety are a thing of the past, and she is thriving, as all parents want for their children. Removing the pressure from her neck changed her entire life.

The same pathways hold true regardless of age. Mental health has come a long way from the stigma of the past but we still have a long way to go. As we learn more about brain function and what a brain needs to be healthy our understanding goes up.

If someone comes to me with a heart that is malfunctioning no one thinks "oh look at Barry with his heart...that guy needs to get it together". Why should brain health be any different? In the case of the heart, we look at the blood flow, we look at the nerve conduction, and we establish where the blockage is located or where the transmission is being interrupted. The same principles apply in the brain. I discussed proper blood flow earlier and we just walked the path to the emotional structures in the brain. A physical issue can, without a doubt, lead to a mental issue. Just as a mental issue can lead to a physical ailment.

How many times have you heard "they had an accident and were never the same"? Personality changes following physical traumas are pretty common. I had a mother bring me her young son and tell me that since he took a hard hit to the head in football he was a completely different kid. He was once loving, easy to deal with, and a great big brother. Since this hit, yelling battles and endless aggravation to his little brother had become their life. Once we corrected his neck we began to see the old personality reemerge.

In the last chapter, I discussed the impact of an upper cervical misalignment on hormones. We can say the same thing here. Dopamine and serotonin levels need to be in proper balance (whether we call these two hormones or neurotransmitters is a topic for a different book) for happiness to occur. These hormones are known as the "happy hormones". Many medications are based around the attempt to balance these chemicals.

Popular drugs like Lexapro, Prozac, Zoloft, etc are in the class of SSRIs. These are based on preventing Serotonin from being reabsorbed. This keeps a higher amount circulating which in theory will increase positive emotions. For some, these medications are magic, but for many, there is little to no benefit and the side effects kick in. BJ Palmer said, "We get sick because something inside goes wrong, we get well because something inside went right". That can't be applied as a blanket statement but it is always wise to fully evaluate the inside before we start adding outside chemicals. You don't have a Lexapro deficiency, if we can equip our bodies to properly regulate themselves we don't have to worry about the negative side effects of adding foreign into our bodies.

Regardless of therapy or medication, if mechanical pressure on the brain stem (an upper cervical misalignment) is disrupting the balance then nothing short of relieving it will give long term improvement. At the very least, it is likely to enhance the therapy and give the medication a better shot at being effective.

CHAPTER 8

HOW DID IT GET THIS WAY?

One of my standard questions in a consultation is "have you ever been in a car accident, any slips or falls, or anytime you might have banged yourself up"? I am hunting for traumas that may have led to a neck injury or misalignment.

I asked a lady we will call Mary this same question. She said she didn't really remember any. I asked if she was sure and she assured me she had not. Her husband's eyes were growing wider the whole time, he finally blurted out "are you kidding me?". He then told me when Mary was 5 years old she was in a car with her sister and mother that was hit by a train.

Patients very commonly forget an accident or fall until I begin to question them. Some walk-in and state a specific day and time that their life changed forever. Either way, it is difficult (almost impossible) to go through life without some type of trauma.

Trauma comes in many forms. The two main ones we want to look at are physical and emotional.

Physical Trauma

Physical is the one we most often think of when we consider trauma. Car accidents, sports injuries, falls and things of that nature. While these are all almost sure to cause an upper neck issue it isn't always a big incident. We talked about the anatomy of the upper neck earlier in the book. A two-ounce bone underneath a twelve-pound head with no locking mechanisms. It doesn't always take a major event.

The physical trauma doesn't always have to be immediately before the symptoms kick in. If you fell off the monkey bars as a kid and jammed your neck it may take years for nerve pressure to begin to show itself.

Sadly, I sit in a consultation far more often than you would imagine hearing that a woman was in an abusive relationship. This type of trauma can be severe and falls into both physical and emotional trauma.

The reality is between birth, learning to walk, running around as a kid and driving on the road it is very difficult to survive it all without the upper neck receiving some level of trauma.

Emotional Trauma

I held (the bone stayed in place) my first Upper Cervical adjustment for one month. I held the second one for three months. Following those, I generally needed to be adjusted every 3-4 months depending on my stress and activity levels.

Years ago I went through a divorce. Most everyone has suffered relationship stress. If you have been through it, you know divorce is at the top of that chart. I suddenly couldn't hold an adjustment for more than two weeks. Sometimes less depending on what was going on.

Think about your physical state when you are under severe stress. Your shoulders feel like they are in your ears, your entire back is tight, your stomach is in knots and energy levels drop dramatically. We know stress can cause heart attacks. This same physical toll can also lead to an upper neck misalignment. All vertebrae have a number of muscles attached to them. If those muscles get tight enough they can shift the bone out of place. Since the top bone is both the smallest and most freely movable it is usually the one to be most affected.

Emotional stress comes in all forms. Job stress, relationships, financial difficulties and all the things that make up our life.

I have checked thousands of spines in my career. As I write this I have found 7 that were free and clear of nerve interference and misalignment. Upper Cervical misalignments are incredibly common because we all suffer trauma in one way or another as we go through life.

CHAPTER 9

WHY HAS THIS NOT BEEN FOUND?

I usually ask patients if they have any prior imaging. MRIs, CT scans, or other scans that show what is going on on the inside. Often they do, but state that the issue wasn't found. My standard response is "that's ok I'm looking for something else".

Patients often arrive in my office in one of two categories.

Category 1 is the group who has been through MRIs, CT scans, endless blood work, and a battery of other tests and the answer always comes back the same...there is nothing wrong with you. At least nothing that explains the current suffering.

Category 2 are the folks who have a diagnosis. They found the answer they were looking for but the conventional forms of treatment have failed. Medications, physical therapy, surgeries and more have all failed to resolve the problem.

The first category begins to wonder if it will ever be found and the second may feel hopeless because it was found but can't be corrected. Either way, by the time they reach me both fear they may "just have to live with it". Even still they sit in my office with the weight of impossibilities on their shoulders and I am often struck by the determined attitude that they will keep searching no matter what.

So many patients are extremely frustrated with their primary care, the neurologist, the pain management doctor and anyone else who has had a hand in their care. I certainly understand the frustration but those people are usually experts at what they do. The problem is they are only as capable as their training. If the issue lies within their training they find both the issue and the solution. If it does not, that is when patients don't have a solution. If you were bitten by a Super Bug while traveling internationally I would refer you out instantly. Being great at what you do also involves knowing when you are the right tool for the job and when you are not.

With UC care, the misalignments we are looking for are small. Often a few millimeters and a couple of degrees. I have been highly trained to find those millimeters and degrees and then correct them. The medical community is looking for severe arthritis, fracture, dislocation, tumors, and things like that. They simply aren't trained or instructed to look for these misalignments.

No matter how hard you look for something you will never find it if you aren't looking in the right place. I have had countless patients with nerve issues in their arms or legs. Traditional thinking is to look at the level of the spine where the nerves exit. At times that is where the problem lies but we have to look at the entire nerve. An impingement at the top will produce a problem wherever that nerve eventually travels whether that is your heart, liver, lungs, arms or legs. The same goes for all of the other conditions I have already discussed. If you can't find your keys on the table by the door you have to start looking everywhere else they could be, under the mail and even in the refrigerator if it has been one of those days. It doesn't make any sense to keep looking on the same table over and over hoping they magically appear.

CHAPTER 10

HOW LONG DOES IT TAKE?

I had terrible teeth as a kid. My parent's insurance likely covered the orthodontist's monthly overhead. I had braces, rubber bands that hooked to the braces and even headgear...you know the things that hook in your mouth and run out around the sides of your face. Thankfully I only had to wear that at night. The point is, it took a lot of work to get my teeth straight because they came in so crooked. I went through all this for 18 months and then wore a retainer at night for many years following. If you think about it, the teeth aren't really the problem, it is the soft tissue around them. That soft tissue takes time to shift and mold into a position that holds the teeth straight.

In the case of an upper cervical injury (and in reality, most misalignments are due to injury whether it was large or small) the soft tissue is the issue. The bones themselves are held in position by the soft tissue around them. The muscles, ligaments, tendons, and other tissues keep our bones and organs where they belong.

The anatomy of the upper neck makes this even more important. From the third bone in the neck to the bottom of the spine there is a disc between each vertebrae. We are all familiar with disc bulges or herniations. The disc is kind of a jelly donut that is glued to the bone above and below. The disc serves as a cushion but also gives strength to the spine. The joints between the vertebrae are interlocking which makes them much harder to injure and misalign.

Where do we have more range of motion? Our head and neck or lower back? Unless you are a contortionist on America's Got Talent the answer is head/neck. The ability to move our head all around like we do requires a very different anatomy. The top two bones in the neck are responsible for a great deal of this movement. They do not have a disc between them and the joints are very flat. This allows a lot more movement but decreases the strength and stability. They are held together by rubber bands. Muscles, ligaments, and tendons are strong but not nearly as strong as a disc and locking joints.

Now that we have examined the anatomy we can get back to our question. How long does it take? The answer is two-part or rather it really is a two-part question. How long does it take to feel better and how long does it take to really heal?

The amount of time to feel better is fairly individual. There are those I call light switches. Adjusting the upper neck is like flipping on the lights and there is instant relief and improvement. Tim is a great example. Tim came in white as a sheet, sweating, and barely able to walk. He was a 10 out of 10 for sciatic pain. If you have ever had sciatica you know it is miserable. Shooting pain in the hip and down the leg. Almost like someone plugged a live electric wire into your leg. Tim had dealt with this on and off for years but this was definitely the worst episode. When he came in, he wasn't very confident that a "neck guy" could solve his problem, but he was desperate.

During the consult, he ended up lying on the floor because that was the only position that wasn't agony. From the examination, I found the second bone in his neck was twisted. This lead to his spine and hips twisting and muscle spasms. The muscle that runs over the top of the sciatic nerve was in a spasm and compressing the nerve. I laid Tim on his side and gently adjusted the second bone and returned it to its proper place. I stepped back and told him to lie there as long as he needed and when he was ready he could stand up. He took a minute or two and stood up. When he did he looked at me across the room with wide eyes. He just stared at me for a bit and finally said, "come on Doc". I will admit I didn't think things were going in a positive direction at this point. Then he said, "this is ridiculous, no way, no freaking way". I finally said Tim you have to let me in on what is going on. He looked at me and said "I have no pain, none at all" he then proceeded to run across the room and bear hug me right into the hall and almost right on the ground. Tim was a light switch. Flip it and bam….results you can see (feel) instantly. This wasn't Tim's last visit and it took us some time for his neck to become stable and adjustments to hold long term which is really the key to the whole story. Feeling great immediately is fantastic but holding the adjustment long enough for the old injury to heal up is the big idea. This is why even for a light switch response it doesn't take just one visit. If we could fix you in one visit we would.

I wish everyone was a light switch but that just isn't the way it works. Like most things, it is a process of time. I am not talking years but sometimes it is weeks or months. On average, patients start to feel relief in the first few weeks, but long term healing takes time. If someone comes to me 20 years after a car accident or fall, it is unrealistic to expect to be fully healed and out the door in a visit or two. The amount of damage, time since injury, lifestyle, and stress levels all factor in. As you saw in my story at the beginning, I was certainly not a light switch.

On the other side of the equation, once you are stable and healed up as long as any additional trauma doesn't occur you can coast in maintenance. Oh, maintenance….why do I have to go back if I am as I said, stable and healed up? Remember a few paragraphs up in Upper Cervical anatomy 101? We talked about how freely moving those bones are and they have a big heavy head on top of them? It is possible, yet highly unlikely that those bones are going to stay in position for the rest of your life without some intervention. What that looks like really depends on the patient and how long they hold an adjustment. If you have someone with a very minor injury and little damage that could be 6 months, maybe even a year. A person with multiple car accidents (for example) may hold a month or two. Just like when you smooth out a piece of crumpled paper it is impossible to get it back to fully smooth again.

Same thing applies, we simply do not have the healthy tissue we once had.

I have been healed since 2006 and I get checked monthly. Not necessarily because I need to be adjusted monthly but just in case. I have no desire to start falling back into the mess I was in years ago. Understanding the potential damage being done by staying out of alignment along with the simplicity of getting properly adjusted I'd rather not assume everything is okay.

CHAPTER 11

I DON'T WANT MY NECK CRACKED

The thought of lying down on your back and having someone grab your head and twist it to one side then the other as your neck cracks like you are stomping branches is a bit scary to most people. I am one of those people. In fact, when I was in chiropractic school, a classmate told me he just wanted to feel my neck. I consented then when I was down there he twisted and adjusted me. I came off the table ready to throw a punch. My point being, I am not a fan. Besides, I don't feel it is necessary and there are better ways to go about it. This is a non-specific adjustment where UC is incredibly precise requiring a minimum amount of pressure and no twisting.

The bones of the neck are smaller than anywhere in the spine and when it comes to the top 2 bones (the upper cervical spine) they are the smallest and most freely movable. It simply doesn't require a big whipping force to align them. It takes precision and exact placement. If we figure out exactly how it is misaligned and where it needs to be placed it takes a slight move to get the job done. The top bone in the neck weighs about 2 ounces. Think about it, if you had something in your hand that weighs two ounces you could blow on it and move it. It doesn't take force to move 2 ounces.

Every person looks different on the outside and the same is true on the inside. The exact shape of the bones and the angles of the joints between them are going to be a little different for everyone. A general shove in a direction is going to require more force and likely not really put the bone back exactly where it needs to be.

With specific x rays, we find the exact misalignment down to a degree or millimeter. This also takes into account the patient's exact anatomy.

Once this is done it takes the lightest touch to restore alignment. This doesn't involve any twisting or popping whatsoever.

The concern with children especially babies is even higher. I have adjusted babies just days old. The amount of pressure used is so light it barely dents the skin. They have tiny bones that are still largely cartilage. It takes the same amount of pressure you could handle on your eyeball to move the bone of a baby.

The best part is with more specific adjustments, not only is it less scary and aggressive, it is also much more effective. This allows the bone to stay in alignment longer and reduces the number of visits needed.

I am fond of saying "if a whiplash got you into this I don't think a whiplash is going to get you out of it". In an Upper Cervical office, you don't have to worry about having a poltergeist type head twist.

CHAPTER 12

WHAT IF I HAVE ALREADY HAD

SPINAL SURGERY?

I had a patient named John come to my office years ago. John worked on new construction and had to crawl in and out of tight spaces for most of his working day. He also had 2 spinal fusions in his neck. He had numbness and tingling in his hands and arms almost constantly, he had constant neck pain, and most days he had a significant headache. John thought he was too far gone to get help but came in to find out. I learned he had 4 vertebrae in a row fused together. Two surgeries over the span of a few years. The 4th through the 7th bones in his neck were literally screwed together. This limited the range of motion in his neck and put a tremendous amount of pressure on his upper neck and upper back. Think about it, 4 of the 7 bones in your neck have to move as one big giant bone. Add in the pressure of constantly crawling around under floors and looking around and you can see why John was miserable. After an exam and x-rays, you could see a giant rotation in the top bone in his neck. I corrected it and after one more adjustment in the week to follow John came in all smiles. The numbness in his arms was practically gone! His neck pain was down from a 7-8 out of10 to a 2 and he hadn't had a headache in 3 days!

By adjusting the top bone (C1 or Atlas) we took the pressure off nerves and restored the range of motion which he was capable of having in spite of his surgeries. The adjustment was safe with no twisting or turning of his fused neck.

There are two types of spinal surgeries that I see most of the time: fusion and decompression.

A fusion is basically a metal plate slapped on the front of two vertebrae and titanium screws drilled into the bone to hold it in place. This type of surgery occurs for several reasons. If a bone is fractured or rendered extremely unstable from an accident; this allows some stability to be returned by fusing the injured bone to a bone above or below that is not injured. At times, such severe degeneration occurs that the decision is made to hook the two damaged bones together as the cushion between them is almost gone.

Increased degeneration above and below a fusion is a common issue following surgery. Once you restrict two bones from independent movement it puts increased stress on the joints and vertebrae above and below.

If you look at a lot of neck x rays, you will notice that the top 3 bones in the neck rarely degenerate and surgeries to this area are rare. In traumatic cases, it is certainly possible for this area to be fractured but in long term wear and tear you just do not see it as often. This means that most anyone who has had a spinal surgery is still a candidate for upper cervical care. The fact that the adjusting does not involve twisting or turning the spine in any way allows for care to be given without worrying about damaging the vertebrae that have already been operated on.

Decompression surgery is the other spinal surgery I see frequently. This occurs when a bone is pressing on a nerve so a portion of the bone is cut out to relieve that pressure. This is most common in the lumbar spine but can be done in the cervical spine. Unfortunately for some, the bone is removed and the symptoms persist. When a case gets to the decompression stage the patient is usually in absolute misery or has lost a considerable amount of function of an arm or leg. Often it is both. The nerve is pinched and if it is a pain referring nerve it is screaming non-stop. If it is a motor nerve then the muscles aren't getting the signal to contract and you lose a significant amount of strength in that limb. It can also be a sensory nerve and in that case numbness or tingling occurs. If the nerve travels to an organ it is impossible for that organ to continue to function normally.

Patients run into trouble when the location of the nerve exiting the spine is either not the area of compression or it wasn't the only area. Remember, all nerves travel from the brain down. Compression at any point can produce the same symptoms. If the top of the neck is pinching that nerve you may still have issues in the affected arm or leg. Surgery is performed but isn't successful and then everyone is left wondering why it didn't work.

I also see patients with very successful decompression surgeries who have other spinal or health issues. In those cases, I stay away from the surgery area but the rest of the spine can certainly be dealt with, and we continue to see improvements and restoration.

Spinal surgery is definitely not something that rules out someone from receiving care. Everyone is a case by case basis but the vast majority of patients I have seen with previous spinal surgeries have had great results. John is still working and feels better than he has in many years. He is certainly living proof of the potential of upper cervical care for these cases.

CHAPTER 13

DEGENERATIVE DISC DISEASE...

IS IT REALLY A DISEASE?

Let's jump back into my story for a minute. When I was 31 and be-gan upper cervical care my neck was a train wreck. I have been in practice since 2009 and have seen thousands of x-rays and I have yet to see a neck in worse shape in anyone under the age of 40. I had very little disc left between C5 and C6 and a bone spur off of C5 that looked like an eagle claw.

When I was in my early 20's a chiropractor took x-rays of my entire spine. He did a very very short report on them but the thing that stuck in my mind was "your spine is in much worse shape than I would have expected". I will readily admit I assumed that was a sales tactic. Yeah, kid, it looks pretty rough you are going to really need me. It turns out he was spot on and being 100% honest. The curve in my neck was com-pletely backwards and the rest of the curves were not much better.

Did I have degenerative disc disease or poor spinal mechanics?

I am going to give you my opinion. It isn't backed by actual research studies or published papers. I am giving it out of looking at spines since 2009 and analyzing tens of thousands of x-rays. I believe there are those who are genetically predisposed to degeneration and those who are not. If I look at my family history, this stands out. On my mom's side, de-generation and spinal issues abound. On my dad's, it doesn't seem to matter how they live or what they do, they all live to an old age and do it well. My great-grandpa was in his 90's tending a garden daily and I would watch him bend almost straight over like he was doing a toe touch to pull a weed. As a 6-year- old I thought that was impressive, now that I am an adult I wonder if he was human.

Unfortunately, I did not win the genetic lottery when it came to degeneration. That is just the way it is but…the real issue was the horrible biomechanics of my neck. The top bone had been knocked forward and left and in my body's attempt to compensate for that bad position, the curve in my neck was backwards.

The curve in the neck should look a bit like a banana with the ends pointing to the left (if you are looking right). If you have a banana near you pick it up and hold it that way. The curve in the upper back (thoracic) should be like the banana with the ends to the right and the lower back curve is the same direction as the neck. The curves should act like shock absorbers to absorb the weight of our head and torso. They compress and expand like a spring as we move and bounce around.

The position of the head on the spine largely determines if these curves are correct or altered. If the head is out in front, the spine will change to compensate for the extra weight out front. If it is tilted to one side or rotated it will also compensate. This compensation leads to altered curves and a stiffening of the spine.

As long as those curves are roughly correct, degeneration doesn't really develop. The joints, the discs, the bones, ligaments, tendons, and muscles all do the job they were designed to do. If the curves straighten or reverse. now we are in trouble.

Rather than work like springs, the weight of the head and torso beat down on the spine day after day. The soft tissue of the discs wears out faster than bone and that space begins to degenerate and get smaller. The ligaments and tendons get inflamed in the areas of the greatest pressure. The bone recognizes this as damage and begins to grow new bone to try to fix it. Now we have bone spurs.

Bone spurs can lead to two big issues. We discussed spinal stenosis in an earlier chapter. Bone spurs that grow into either the spinal canal or the space where nerves exit the spine can create stenosis. A spur that has grown large enough can start to put pressure on either the spinal cord or spinal nerves. You do not want to be in a situation for either of those to occur. The other possible outcome is a spur that grows so large off the front of the vertebrae that it eventually meets with a spur from the bone above or below and they grow together. A bony bridge develops and those two vertebrae are essentially fused together, much like when a plate is applied to the bones in a fusion surgery. Both of these processes take time. By time I mean years and often decades.

If the disc space degenerates and gets smaller this can also lead to stenosis. The space between the bones allows the spinal nerves to exit the spinal canal and into the rest of the body. If this space gets smaller because the cushion between the discs shrink, we can get nerve pressure.

Back to genetics, I believe the rate of degeneration, once proper positioning is lost, depends greatly on that person's genetics. I have seen 40-year-olds with pretty severe degeneration and 80-year-olds with very little. While we can't do much about that side of things, preserving proper mechanics is relatively easy. If the bones of the spine, especially those right under the head, are in proper position (and moving correctly) the spine will remain flexible and maintain proper curves.

If that is the case, degeneration will not really be a factor affecting health.

While we are on the subject...if the spine is imbalanced and the weight of the torso isn't evenly balanced it is likely that the hips and knees will also degenerate faster. If one side is carrying 10 or 20 lbs more weight because the spine has shifted then the knee or hip on that side will certainly wear out faster than it should. Just like bad alignment in your car will wear your tires unevenly the same goes for the joints in the body.

Let's get back to me (who doesn't like talking about themselves). Remember I had a spur that looked like an eagle claw? That spur is almost gone now. Once the abnormal pressure is relieved from the ligaments and tendons the inflammation disappears. When there is no inflammation, there is no need for the extra bone and the body reabsorbs it. Think about a callus on your hand. If you are doing repetitive labor the body builds up a callus to thicken the hand and protect it. If you stop doing that activity and no longer need the callus, the body stops creating a callus. The same principle applies here.

Unfortunately, some bones or discs are too far gone to save but that doesn't mean the rest of the spine can't be salvaged. The sooner you stop these negative processes, the better you can reverse a great deal of damage given proper mechanics and time.

This is one of the many reasons I encourage parents to get their kids checked. If we prevent the spine from being in a bad position when they are young, they may never have to deal with the issues many older people fight.

CHAPTER 14

IS UPPER CERVICAL CARE FOR ME?

Honest answer...I can't tell you for sure without first examining you. I can tell you I have checked thousands of people and so far I have found 7 without an Upper Cervical misalignment. I can also tell you getting into the world isn't always easy. Difficult labor, c-sections, having to pull to get the baby out. Then learning to walk is a bobble fest with many falls and potential headbangs. Once a kid is mobile they usually run their head into a million things. Going through life we all have slips and falls. Car accidents are fairly common. My point being, there are a multitude of opportunities in an average life to bang your neck up and create a misalignment, impede nerve function and cause dysfunction.

It may be a big incident you can point to and say , "yep that's when it all went downhill" or something that seemed minor but in reality, was the beginning of the downward slide. Often patients tell me they had a car wreck but went to the hospital, had x-rays, and everything was negative. The reality is, ER docs are looking for fractures, ligament tears, the big stuff. They don't have the training or time to analyze millimeter misalignments that may eventually rob you of your health.

It was December 10th, 2012. I was closing my first office. We had told patients we would be in the office until 12pm if anyone wanted to pick up records. Around 11:45 a guy we will call Ron walked in. Ron was a very special patient. He had helped to open my eyes to what can be possible through Upper Cervical chiropractic care.

When Ron first came in, he told me he wasn't sure if he should even be there. He had end-stage liver failure. He was on the donor list but due to age and some other factors, it was highly unlikely he would move to the top of the list. Everything had been tried with no result and he was now planning on living life to the fullest as long as he could, then it would be over. He came in because a good friend and longtime UC patient told him it was worth a shot.

I told him I had no idea if I could help him but we would try. I will be honest with you. I had very little confidence in the outcome. I had heard incredible stories from other UC docs but I was new in practice and this seemed over my head, maybe the death diagnosis had intimidated me. It was around May of 2010. Over the next 6 months (his expected time left) I only adjusted the top bone in his neck a total of 3 times. He was a terribly unreliable patient. (When you are on a death clock appointments lose importance).

Ron went in every few months to have his liver enzymes checked and to recertify for the donor list. We hit the 6-month mark and Ron went to get his levels checked. The doctors looked at them and ran a second round of tests. Funny thing was they were normal. The second round of tests confirmed the first. His liver was functioning completely normal.

Ron came in to tell me the news and I just stood there in disbelief, This man was literally dying. Then we both shed a few tears and shared a giant hug. His life was restored because nerve function was restored.

Back to 11:45 and the last patient of the practice. Ron walked in smiling. I commented on how great it was he ended up being the final patient. He had planned it all along. It was a special moment for all of us as we joined hands and he prayed for the future of all of us. He walked out of the door and I was reminded of what was possible when you allow the body to do what it was designed to do. Heal.

Before you call the sheriff to run my snake oil wagon out of town, as the great chiropractor Jim Sigafoose said: "if the body can create disease it can cure it." I have witnessed the truth in that statement countless times in my practice.

I would like to tell you every story ends with seemingly miraculous re-sults. While I will testify many do, it isn't a guarantee. The chances of restoring health are always better with a nervous system free of interfer-ence.

I don't know if UC is your miracle. I haven't met you and I don't know what you are dealing with. I have thousands of testimonials I have wit-nessed which continue to confirm the life-changing power and benefits of specific chiropractic care done through Upper Cervical adjustments. I know it was mine. I know it was Rons'. I sure hope it is yours but I can't make promises. I will, however, leave you with one question.

What if...???

CHAPTER 15

HOW DO I FIND AN UPPER CERVICAL CHIROPRACTOR?

I f you read this and do not live in SWFL you may be wondering where do you go and how do find an Upper Cervical chiropractor near you.

There are several directories you can search. The ones I go to most often are:

www.uppercervicalcare.com

www.upcspine.com

www.blairchiropractic.com

nucca.org

orthospinology.org

These do not list every single UC office in existence but will cover most of them.

When calling an office there are two main questions you can ask to ensure you are getting Upper Cervical Chiropractic.

Do you take x-rays? Any legitimate Upper Cervical doctor takes precision x-rays. As we discussed earlier, the upper neck requires precision in both analysis and correction.

What technique does the doctor use? Within the world of Upper Cervical, there are a number of different techniques. We are all after the same result, realigning the upper neck. There are just variations on how the x-rays are taken and how the adjustment is delivered.

The main techniques are:

- Blair Upper Cervical
- Knee Chest
- Toggle Recoil
- NUCCA
- Atlas Orthogonal
- Orthospinology
- Grostic

This is not all known techniques but the most popular. Ultimately the technique will be named. If they cannot provide a technique name you may want to look elsewhere.

I can tell you from personal and patient experience it is worth a bit of travel if that is required. Upper Cervical can be that powerful. I have had patients fly in from other countries and spend a month in a hotel. Others make a days drive for this care. Your health is worth the effort!

AUTHOR BIO

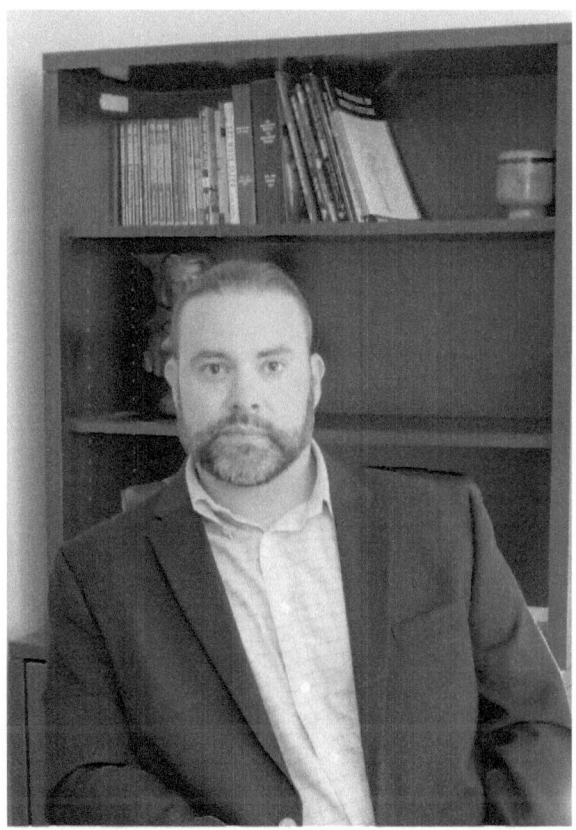

Dr. Lee Angle is a graduate of Sherman College of Chiropractic with a B.S. from Virginia Tech. He has been practicing Upper Cervical Chiropractic for over a decade and has been featured on Fox television, Fox radio and ESPN radio speaking about the benefits of proper neck alignment. Dr. Angle has helped patients from all over the world to restore their health from a wide variety of conditions.

www.DrLeeAngle.com

www.ingramcontent.com/pod-product-compliance
Lightning Source LLC
Chambersburg PA
CBHW021506210526
45463CB00002B/916